Heart's Electric Symphony: Understanding Cardiac Arrhythmias

By

Prajwal Kadam

ISBN: 9798862330311

Disclaimer: While writing this book, The assistance of large language models (LLMs) has been utilized in order to generate a very small proportion of the content in the book. However, a significant portion of the book has also been written manually by referring to academic journals, textbooks, and other reliable sources. Every effort has been made to ensure that the information presented in this book which has been written with the help of LLMs, is accurate and up-to-date. All the sources have been cited appropriately.

About Ioncure

Ioncure is a 360 degrees wellness company, which puts services ahead of profits. In addition to cutting edge knowledge of our very talented team, our commitment to citizen science, education, and interdisciplinary approaches sets us aside. We are not just early adopters of technology, a significant portion of Ioncure's effort is spent developing 4th industrial revolution technology.

We are a company with four pillars: artificial intelligence, life science, citizen science, and education, and we believe that one shoe fits all approaches to healthcare, education, and shelter should belong to museums. We are here to find new medicines, supplements, and instruments, which are designed for the individuals. We look forward to making the world a better place through your support and becoming a part of the Ioncure family.

We do not confine our interest in healthcare to merely medicines or supplements. Anything, and everything that can contribute to improved wellness of an individual is our concern. Ioncure is the name of revolution, which aims to transform our society through wellness, and it is not just another business.

Sukant Khurana, Founder and CEO,

Ioncure Tech Pvt Ltd.

Contents

Chapter 1: Life and healthcare in West Bengal

Introduction to West Bengal's natural beauty, biodiversity, and geology

West Bengal, located in the eastern region of India, boasts of a rich natural beauty, diverse biodiversity, and unique geology. The state is blessed with a vast coastline, with the Bay of Bengal to its south, and the mighty Himalayas to its north. The Sunderbans, the largest mangrove forest in the world, is a UNESCO World Heritage Site and home to the majestic Royal Bengal Tiger. The state also has a rich floral and faunal diversity with several national parks, wildlife sanctuaries, and bird sanctuaries, including the Gorumara National Park, Neora Valley National Park, and Singalila National Park. The state's geological features are equally fascinating, with the Darjeeling hills known for its tea gardens, and the Purulia district famous for its red soil and rolling topography. Overall, West Bengal is a treasure trove of natural beauty, biodiversity, and geology, making it a must-visit destination for nature enthusiasts and adventurers.

Tourist attractions in West Bengal

West Bengal is a state rich in culture, history, and natural beauty, with many attractions that draw visitors from all over the world

1. The Sundarbans: The largest mangrove forest in the world, home to the Royal Bengal Tiger and a UNESCO World Heritage Site.

2. Darjeeling: Famous for its tea plantations, scenic beauty, and the Darjeeling Himalayan Railway, a UNESCO World Heritage Site.

3. Kolkata: The cultural capital of India, with colonial architecture, bustling markets, and delicious street food.

4. Victoria Memorial: An iconic museum in Kolkata, dedicated to the memory of Queen Victoria and showcasing a collection of rare artifacts and paintings.

5. Bishnupur: A historic town known for its terracotta temples, intricate weaving, and pottery.

6. Digha: A popular seaside resort town, known for its beautiful beaches, amusement parks, and seafood.

7. Shantiniketan: A serene town known for its cultural and educational heritage, and the home of Nobel laureate Rabindranath Tagore.

8. Sunderban Tiger Reserve: A national park and UNESCO World Heritage Site, known for its rich biodiversity, including the Royal Bengal Tiger.

9. Murshidabad: A historic town known for its palaces, museums, and the Hazarduari Palace, a unique 108-room palace.

10. Kalimpong: A charming hill station known for its scenic beauty, colonial architecture, and Buddhist monasteries.

Living in West Bengal

Living in West Bengal is an experience like no other. The state is known for its rich culture, traditions, and warm hospitality. The people of West Bengal are known for their love of literature, music, art, and food, and you will find a vibrant cultural scene wherever you go. The streets of Kolkata are bustling with activity, and you can always find something to do or see, whether it's watching a play, attending a concert, or exploring the city's many markets.

One of the most striking things about living in West Bengal is the diversity of the state. From the lush green forests of the Sunderbans to the tea plantations of Darjeeling, the state has something to offer for everyone. The people of West Bengal are proud of their cultural heritage, and you will find a strong sense of community wherever you go. Whether it's celebrating Durga Puja, the state's most important festival, or simply gathering with friends and family for a meal, there is always a reason to come together and celebrate.

Despite its many charms, living in West Bengal can also be challenging at times. The state faces a range of issues, including poverty, environmental degradation, and political instability. However, the people of West Bengal are resilient, and there is a strong sense of solidarity among the community. Overall, living in West Bengal is a unique and rewarding experience, full of rich culture, natural beauty, and warm hospitality.

History of West Bengal

West Bengal has a rich and complex history that spans thousands of years.

1. Ancient History: West Bengal has a rich ancient history dating back to the Vedic period. The region was ruled by various kingdoms, including the Mauryas, Guptas, and Pala dynasties.

2. Islamic Rule: The region came under the rule of the Delhi Sultanate in the 13th century and later the Mughal Empire in the 16th century. The state saw the rise of the independent Bengal Nawabs in the 18th century.

3. British Rule: The British East India Company gained control of Bengal in 1757 after the Battle of Plassey. The region became the center of British colonial administration, with Kolkata as its capital. The region saw significant political, social, and economic changes during this period.

4. Partition of Bengal: In 1905, the British government partitioned Bengal into two administrative divisions, sparking widespread protests and the Swadeshi Movement. The partition was later revoked in 1911.

5. Post-Independence: West Bengal became a part of independent India in 1947. The state has seen significant political and social changes, including the Naxalite movement and the rise of the Left Front government, which governed the state from 1977 to 2011. The state has also been a hub of cultural and intellectual activity, producing notable figures such as Rabindranath Tagore, Satyajit Ray, and Amartya Sen.

Cities of West Bengal

The state is home to many cities, each with its own story to tell. Each city in Louisiana has a unique history and culture that contributes to the state's overall identity. From the Creole cuisine of New Orleans to the Cajun culture of Lafayette,

Louisiana's cities are full of rich history and traditions that make it a special place to visit and explore.

1. **Kolkata:** The capital city of West Bengal and the cultural hub of the state. Kolkata is known for its colonial architecture, museums, art galleries, and street food. It is also home to several landmarks, such as the Victoria Memorial and Howrah Bridge.

2. **Darjeeling:** A picturesque hill station located in the foothills of the Himalayas. Darjeeling is famous for its tea plantations, scenic beauty, and the Darjeeling Himalayan Railway, a UNESCO World Heritage Site.

3. **Siliguri:** A bustling city located in the north of West Bengal, near the border with Nepal and Bhutan. Siliguri is an important commercial hub, and also serves as a gateway to the northeastern states of India.

4. **Asansol:** A major industrial city located in the western part of West Bengal. Asansol is known for its coal mines, steel plants, and thermal power plants.

5. **Durgapur:** Another major industrial city located in the eastern part of West Bengal. Durgapur is known for its steel and alloy plants, and is also an important educational and cultural center.

6. **Haldia:** A port city located on the banks of the Hooghly River, in the southern part of West Bengal. Haldia is an important industrial hub, with several major companies having operations in the area.

7. **Malda:** A historic city located in the northern part of West Bengal, near the border with Bangladesh. Malda is known for its historic landmarks, such as the Adina Mosque and the Gour-Pandua archaeological site.

8. **Bankura:** A town located in the western part of West Bengal, known for its temples, museums, and the Susunia Hills, a popular trekking destination.

9. **Purulia:** A district located in the western part of West Bengal, known for its natural beauty, tribal culture, and historic landmarks, such as the Baghmundi Fort and the Cheliama temple.

10. **Krishnanagar:** A town located in the eastern part of West Bengal, known for its historic landmarks, such as the Rajbari Palace and the Bethuadahari Wildlife Sanctuary.

Culture of West Bengal

West Bengal has a rich and diverse culture that is reflected in its art, music, literature, food, festivals, and traditions. The state is known for its vibrant cultural scene, which includes classical and folk music, dance, theater, and cinema. The famous Bengali poet, Rabindranath Tagore, is a symbol of the state's cultural heritage and is widely celebrated for his contributions to literature, music, and art. The state is also known for its culinary traditions, with famous dishes such as the Kolkata-style biryani, fish curry, and sweets such as rasgulla and sandesh.

One of the most significant aspects of West Bengal's culture is its festivals and traditions. Durga Puja, the state's biggest festival, is celebrated with great pomp and show, and brings together people from all walks of life. Other important festivals include Diwali, Eid, Christmas, and Holi, all of which are celebrated with great enthusiasm and vigor. The state is also known for its cultural diversity, with people of different religions, languages, and ethnic backgrounds living together in harmony.

Overall, West Bengal's culture is a unique blend of tradition and modernity, reflecting the state's rich history and diverse cultural influences. The state's people are proud of their cultural heritage and continue to celebrate it through art, music, literature, and festivals. West Bengal's culture is an integral part of its identity, and has played a significant role in shaping the state's character and identity.

MajorHospitals in West Bengal

1. **Apollo Gleneagles Hospital:** One of the largest private hospitals in Kolkata, Apollo Gleneagles Hospital is known for its world-class facilities and expertise in various medical specialties. The hospital has over 700 beds and offers services such as cardiology, neurology, orthopedics, oncology, and gastroenterology.

2. **Medica Superspecialty Hospital**: Another leading private hospital in Kolkata, Medica Superspecialty Hospital has state-of-the-art facilities and a team of highly qualified doctors and healthcare professionals. The hospital offers a wide range of medical services, including cardiology, neurology, urology, orthopedics, and pediatrics.

3. **AMRI Hospitals:** With three locations in Kolkata, AMRI Hospitals is a leading chain of hospitals in West Bengal. The hospitals offer a wide range of medical services, including cardiology, oncology, neurology, orthopedics, and gastroenterology. The hospital also has a dedicated department for emergency and trauma care.

4. **Tata Medical Center:** Located in Kolkata, Tata Medical Center is a renowned hospital that specializes in cancer care and treatment. The hospital has state-of-the-art facilities and a team of highly skilled oncologists and healthcare professionals. The hospital also conducts research in cancer treatment and offers various clinical trials.

5. **Institute of Postgraduate Medical Education and Research (IPGMER):** A government-run hospital located in Kolkata, IPGMER is a leading medical institution in West Bengal. The hospital offers services in various medical specialties, including cardiology, neurology, orthopedics, and pediatrics.

Health-related non-profit organizations in West Bengal

1. **Indian Cancer Society (ICS):** The ICS is a non-profit organization that works towards creating awareness about cancer prevention, early detection, and treatment. The organization provides cancer screening and diagnostic services, and also supports cancer patients and their families.

2. **CINI:** Child in Need Institute (CINI) is a non-profit organization that works towards improving the health and wellbeing of women and children in West Bengal. The organization provides healthcare services, education, and nutrition support to children, as well as support for maternal and reproductive health.

3. **The Calcutta Rescue:** The Calcutta Rescue is a non-profit organization that provides medical and social support to the homeless, destitute, and marginalized communities in Kolkata. The organization operates a mobile medical unit that provides primary healthcare services to people living in slums and on the streets.

4. **HelpAge India:** HelpAge India is a non-profit organization that works towards improving the health and wellbeing of senior citizens in India. The organization provides healthcare services, support for social and economic empowerment, and advocacy for the rights of elderly people.

5. **The Leprosy Mission:** The Leprosy Mission is a non-profit organization that works towards the prevention and treatment of leprosy in India. The organization provides medical and rehabilitation services to people affected by leprosy, as well as advocacy for their rights and inclusion in society.

Government bodies for general health in West Bengal

The government bodies work together to ensure that the residents of West Bengal have access to quality healthcare services and that healthcare professionals in the state are held to high standards of practice.

1. **SSKM Hospital:** Also known as the Seth Sukhlal Karnani Memorial Hospital, it is one of the oldest and largest government hospitals in West Bengal. Located in Kolkata, it offers services in various medical specialties, including cardiology, neurology, urology, and gastroenterology.

2. **Calcutta Medical College and Hospital:** Established in 1835, the Calcutta Medical College and Hospital is the second oldest medical college in India. It offers services in various medical specialties, including cardiology, neurology, orthopaedics, and paediatrics.

3. **North Bengal Medical College and Hospital:** Located in Siliguri, North Bengal Medical College and Hospital is a government-run hospital that offers medical services in various specialties, including cardiology, neurology, orthopaedics, and paediatrics.

4. **RG Kar Medical College and Hospital:** A government-run hospital located in Kolkata, RG Kar Medical College and Hospital offers medical services in various specialties, including cardiology, neurology, orthopaedics, and

paediatrics. The hospital is also a leading center for medical education and research.

5. **Midnapore Medical College and Hospital:** A government-run hospital located in Midnapore, it offers medical services in various specialties, including cardiology, neurology, orthopaedics, and paediatrics. The hospital is also a leading center for medical education and research in the region.

Government health programs and initiatives in West Bengal

1. **Swasthya Sathi**: A flagship health insurance scheme launched by the Government of West Bengal in 2016, Swasthya Sathi provides cashless health insurance cover of up to Rs. 5 lakhs per family per year to the citizens of the state.

2. **Chief Minister's Comprehensive Health Insurance Scheme:** This scheme aims to provide comprehensive health insurance cover to the poor and marginalized sections of society in West Bengal.

3. **Mamata Banerjee Swasthya Sathi scheme:** Launched in 2021, this scheme provides free healthcare services to the people of West Bengal through a network of government hospitals and health centers.

4. **Mental Health Program:** The Government of West Bengal has launched a mental health program to provide access to mental healthcare services to the people of the state. The program includes training of healthcare professionals, community awareness campaigns, and setting up of mental health clinics.

5. **State AIDS Prevention and Control Society:** The West Bengal State AIDS Prevention and Control Society is a government-run program that aims to

prevent the spread of HIV/AIDS in the state. The program includes awareness campaigns, free testing and treatment, and support services for people living with HIV/AIDS.

6. **Janani Shishu Suraksha Karyakram:** A government-run program that provides free maternity and child healthcare services to the women and children of West Bengal.

Chapter 2: Understanding Cardiac Rhythm

Cardiac rhythm refers to the synchronized pattern of electrical impulses that regulate the contractions of the heart muscles. It is the rhythmic coordination between the heart's electrical system and its mechanical function that allows for the effective pumping of blood throughout the body. The normal cardiac rhythm, known as sinus rhythm, is characterized by a regular and coordinated sequence of depolarization and repolarization events. These electrical signals originate from the sinoatrial (SA) node, the natural pacemaker of the heart, and travel through specialized pathways to ensure the sequential contraction of the atria and ventricles.

Understanding and analyzing cardiac rhythm is vital in diagnosing and managing various heart conditions, as deviations from the normal rhythm can indicate underlying abnormalities or arrhythmias that may require medical intervention. In addition to the normal sinus rhythm, there are various other cardiac rhythms that can occur due to different factors or conditions. These include atrial rhythms, ventricular rhythms, and conduction abnormalities. Atrial rhythms involve abnormalities in the electrical signals originating from the atria, which can result in irregular or rapid heartbeats. Ventricular rhythms, on the other hand, involve abnormalities in the electrical signals originating from the ventricles, leading to irregular and potentially life-threatening arrhythmias. Conduction abnormalities refer to disruptions in the transmission of electrical signals through the heart's conduction system, which can result in delays or blocks in the conduction pathway.

Understanding and interpreting cardiac rhythms is achieved through the use of electrocardiography (ECG). An ECG records the electrical activity of the heart and provides a visual representation of the cardiac rhythm. It consists of a series of waveforms and intervals that correspond to the different phases of the cardiac cycle. By analyzing the ECG tracings, healthcare professionals can identify abnormalities, such as irregular rhythms, conduction disturbances, or signs of ischemia or infarction.

Accurate interpretation of cardiac rhythms is crucial for diagnosing and managing various heart conditions. It allows healthcare providers to determine the appropriate treatment strategies, whether it involves medication, interventions, or further diagnostic tests. Moreover, monitoring changes in cardiac rhythm over time can help evaluate the effectiveness of treatment interventions and assess the overall cardiac health of the patient.

Overall, a comprehensive understanding of cardiac rhythm and the ability to interpret ECG tracings are essential skills for healthcare professionals involved in cardiology and critical care. It enables them to identify and address any abnormalities promptly, thereby promoting optimal heart function and improving patient outcomes.

Chapter 3: Introduction to Electrocardiography (ECG)

Electrocardiography, commonly known as ECG or EKG, is a diagnostic tool used to assess the electrical activity of the heart. It provides valuable information about the heart's rhythm, rate, and any potential abnormalities. ECG plays a crucial role in diagnosing various heart conditions, guiding treatment decisions, and monitoring patients' cardiac health. This article aims to provide a comprehensive overview of the basics of ECG, including its purpose, procedure, and interpretation.

Purpose of ECG:

The primary purpose of an ECG is to detect and evaluate abnormalities in the heart's electrical activity. It can help diagnose conditions such as arrhythmias, ischemic heart disease, myocardial infarction, electrolyte imbalances, and structural abnormalities. ECG is a non-invasive and cost-effective test that provides valuable information about the heart's overall function and assists in the management of cardiac patients.

Procedure:

During an ECG procedure, small, adhesive electrodes are placed on specific areas of the patient's chest, arms, and legs. These electrodes detect the electrical signals generated by the heart and transmit them to the ECG machine. The machine then converts these signals into a graphical representation known as an ECG tracing or ECG strip.

Interpretation:

Interpreting an ECG requires a systematic approach and understanding of the various components and intervals observed on the ECG strip. The most common features of an ECG include:

P Wave: Represents atrial depolarization, indicating the initiation of the heart's electrical impulse.

PR Interval: Measures the time between atrial depolarization and ventricular depolarization, representing the delay in electrical conduction through the atrioventricular (AV) node.

QRS Complex: Represents ventricular depolarization, indicating the contraction of the ventricles.

ST Segment: Represents the interval between ventricular depolarization and repolarization, providing information about myocardial oxygenation and ischemia.

T Wave: Represents ventricular repolarization, indicating the relaxation and recovery phase of the ventricles.

To accurately interpret an ECG, healthcare professionals analyze the rhythm, rate, and morphology of the waveforms, as well as the intervals and segments. Abnormalities in these ECG components can indicate underlying cardiac conditions or rhythm disturbances.

Clinical Applications:

ECG has numerous clinical applications and is widely used in various healthcare settings. Some of the key clinical applications of ECG include:

Diagnosis: ECG helps in diagnosing various heart conditions and differentiating between different types of arrhythmias.

Risk Stratification: ECG findings can assist in assessing the risk of cardiovascular events, such as myocardial infarction or sudden cardiac death.

Treatment Guidance: ECG findings guide the selection of appropriate treatment strategies, such as medication, cardioversion, or invasive interventions like cardiac catheterization.

Monitoring: ECG monitoring allows continuous assessment of a patient's cardiac rhythm and detects any changes or abnormalities over time.

Limitations and Considerations:

While ECG is a valuable diagnostic tool, it does have limitations and considerations that should be taken into account. Some key points to consider include:

Single Snapshot: ECG provides a snapshot of the heart's electrical activity at a specific moment. It may not capture transient or intermittent abnormalities, requiring additional monitoring techniques.

Operator Skill: Interpreting an ECG requires training and expertise. Misinterpretation can lead to false-positive or false-negative findings.

Technical Artifacts: Various factors, such as patient movement, improper electrode placement, or electrical interference, can produce artifacts that may affect the accuracy of the ECG.

Limited Diagnostic Scope: While ECG is a valuable tool, it may not detect all types of cardiac abnormalities. Additional diagnostic tests, such as echocardiography or stress testing, may be required for a comprehensive evaluation.

Chapter 4: Cardiac Arrhythmias

Cardiac Arrhythmias: An introduction

Cardiac arrhythmias are a group of disorders that affect the electrical system of the heart, resulting in abnormal heart rhythms. These disorders are prevalent in West Bengal, and their incidence is on the rise due to a variety of factors, including changes in lifestyle, increased longevity, and advances in medical technology.

This book aims to provide a comprehensive overview of cardiac arrhythmias in West Bengal, with a focus on their diagnosis, management, and prevention. It is intended for healthcare professionals, patients, and anyone interested in learning more about this complex and often life-threatening condition.

The book is divided into 15 chapters, each covering a specific aspect of cardiac arrhythmias in West Bengal. The first few chapters provide an introduction to the topic, including an overview of cardiac arrhythmias, their epidemiology, and the different types of arrhythmias that can occur.

Subsequent chapters delve into the causes, risk factors, and diagnostic methods for cardiac arrhythmias, as well as the various treatment options available, such as medication, catheter ablation, and pacemaker implantation. The book also covers surgical procedures for cardiac arrhythmias and includes a chapter on living with cardiac arrhythmias, providing coping strategies and support for patients.

Prevention and lifestyle modification for cardiac arrhythmias are also discussed, as well as advances in the management of these disorders and future directions for research in West Bengal.

Cardiac arrhythmias are a group of disorders that affect the heart's electrical system, leading to abnormal heart rhythms. These disorders can cause a range of symptoms, including palpitations, dizziness, shortness of breath, and even fainting or sudden cardiac arrest.

The heart's electrical system consists of a network of specialized cells that generate and conduct electrical impulses throughout the heart, controlling its rhythm and rate. In a healthy heart, these impulses are generated and conducted in a coordinated manner, resulting in a normal heart rhythm. However, in people with cardiac arrhythmias, this process is disrupted, leading to abnormal heart rhythms.

Chapter 5. Types of Cardiac Arrhythmias

Cardiac arrhythmias can be broadly classified into two categories: tachyarrhythmias and bradyarrhythmias. Tachyarrhythmias are characterized by a heart rate that is too fast, while bradyarrhythmias are characterized by a heart rate that is too slow.

There are several types of cardiac arrhythmias, each with its own unique characteristics and clinical implications.

Some of the most common types of tachyarrhythmias include:

1. Atrial fibrillation: A rapid, irregular heartbeat that can lead to blood clots and stroke

2. Supraventricular tachycardia: A rapid heartbeat that originates above the ventricles.

3. Ventricular tachycardia: A rapid heartbeat that originates in the ventricles and can be life-threatening.

4. Atrial flutter: A rapid, regular heartbeat that originates in the atria.

5. Wolff-Parkinson-White syndrome: An abnormal electrical pathway in the heart that can cause rapid heartbeats.

Some of the most common types of bradyarrhythmias include:

1. Sinus bradycardia: A slow heart rate that originates from the sinus node.

6. Atrioventricular block: A disruption in the electrical impulses between the atria and ventricles.

7. Sick sinus syndrome: A condition where the sinus node does not function properly, leading to slow heart rates.

Chapter 6: Epidemiology of Cardiac Arrhythmias in West Bengal

Cardiac arrhythmias are a significant public health problem in West Bengal, with a high prevalence and incidence rate. According to a study published in the Indian Journal of Medical Research, the prevalence of cardiac arrhythmias in West Bengal is around 4.8%, which is higher than the national average of 3.5%.

The incidence of cardiac arrhythmias is also increasing in West Bengal due to various factors such as an aging population, an increase in lifestyle diseases, and improved diagnostic techniques. Several studies have reported that the prevalence and incidence of cardiac arrhythmias are higher in urban areas compared to rural areas.

Atrial fibrillation is the most common type of cardiac arrhythmia in West Bengal, accounting for around 50% of cases. Other common types of arrhythmias include supraventricular tachycardia, ventricular tachycardia, and atrial flutter. The incidence of sudden cardiac death due to ventricular arrhythmias is also higher in West Bengal compared to other parts of India.

The risk factors for cardiac arrhythmias in West Bengal are similar to those observed in other parts of the world. These include age, hypertension, diabetes, obesity, smoking, and a family history of cardiac arrhythmias. The incidence of cardiac arrhythmias is also higher in patients with structural heart diseases such as coronary artery disease, valvular heart disease, and congenital heart disease.

Chapter 7: Causes and Risk Factors of Cardiac Arrhythmias in West Bengal

The causes of cardiac arrhythmias in West Bengal are multifactorial and often complex. Some of the common causes of cardiac arrhythmias in West Bengal include:

- Structural heart diseases such as coronary artery disease, valvular heart disease, and congenital heart disease.

- Hypertension, diabetes, and other lifestyle diseases.

- Medications such as beta-blockers, calcium channel blockers, and anti-arrhythmic drugs.

- Electrolyte imbalances such as low potassium or magnesium levels.

- Substance abuse such as alcohol, cocaine, and amphetamines.

The risk factors for cardiac arrhythmias in West Bengal are similar to those observed in other parts of the world. These include:

- Age: The risk of cardiac arrhythmias increases with age.

- Hypertension: High blood pressure can increase the risk of cardiac arrhythmias.

- Diabetes: High blood sugar levels can damage the heart and lead to arrhythmias.

- Obesity: Excess weight puts a strain on the heart and increases the risk of arrhythmias.

- Smoking: Nicotine and other chemicals in tobacco smoke can damage the heart and increase the risk of arrhythmias.

- Family history: A family history of cardiac arrhythmias or sudden cardiac death can increase the risk of arrhythmias.

Chapter 8: Symptoms of Cardiac Arrhythmias

The symptoms of cardiac arrhythmias can vary depending on the type and severity of the arrhythmia. Some of the common symptoms of cardiac arrhythmias include:

- Palpitations: A sensation of an irregular or fast heartbeat.

- Shortness of breath: Difficulty breathing or feeling breathless.

- Chest pain or discomfort: A feeling of pressure or tightness in the chest.

- Fatigue: Feeling tired or weak.

- Dizziness or lightheadedness: Feeling faint or unsteady.

- Syncope: A sudden loss of consciousness.

In some cases, cardiac arrhythmias may not cause any symptoms and may only be detected during a routine medical examination or electrocardiogram (ECG).

Chapter 9: Diagnosis of Cardiac Arrhythmias

The diagnosis of cardiac arrhythmias in West Bengal involves a thorough medical history and physical examination, followed by various diagnostic tests. Some of the common diagnostic tests for cardiac arrhythmias include:

- Electrocardiogram (ECG): A test that records the electrical activity of the heart and can detect abnormal heart rhythms.

- Holter monitor: A portable device that records the heart's electrical activity for 24-48 hours to detect intermittent arrhythmias.

- Event monitor: A portable device that records the heart's electrical activity for up to 30 days to detect infrequent arrhythmias.

- Echocardiogram: A test that uses sound waves to create images of the heart and can detect structural abnormalities.

- Cardiac catheterization: A procedure that involves inserting a catheter into a blood vessel and guiding it to the heart to detect blockages or other abnormalities.

- Electrophysiological study (EPS): A test that involves inserting catheters into the heart to measure the electrical signals and locate the origin of the arrhythmia.

Chapter 10: Treatment of Cardiac Arrhythmias

The treatment of cardiac arrhythmias in West Bengal depends on the type and severity of the arrhythmia. Some of the common treatments for cardiac arrhythmias include:

- Medications: Anti-arrhythmic drugs such as beta-blockers, calcium channel blockers, and digoxin can be used to control the heart rate and rhythm.

- Cardioversion: A procedure that uses an electric shock or medication to restore a normal heart rhythm.

- Ablation: A procedure that uses catheters to destroy small areas of heart tissue that are causing the arrhythmia.

- Implantable devices: Pacemakers and implantable cardioverter defibrillators (ICDs) can be used to control the heart rate and rhythm or prevent sudden cardiac death.

- Surgery: In some cases, surgery may be required to correct structural abnormalities or damage to the heart.

Chapter 11: Prevention of Cardiac Arrhythmias

Preventing cardiac arrhythmias in West Bengal involves making healthy lifestyle choices and managing underlying medical conditions.

Some of the ways to prevent cardiac arrhythmias include:

- Maintaining a healthy weight and eating a balanced diet.

- Exercising regularly and staying physically active.

- Quitting smoking and avoiding secondhand smoke.

- Managing underlying medical conditions such as high blood pressure, diabetes, and sleep apnea.

- Limiting alcohol and caffeine intake.

- Managing stress through relaxation techniques, exercise, or counseling.

Chapter 12: Cardiac Arrhythmias and COVID-19

The COVID-19 pandemic has brought new challenges to the management of cardiac arrhythmias in West Bengal. Some studies have shown that COVID-19 can cause cardiac arrhythmias in patients with or without pre-existing heart disease. Additionally, the use of certain medications for COVID-19 treatment can interact with anti-arrhythmic drugs and increase the risk of arrhythmias.

Therefore, it is important for patients with cardiac arrhythmias to take extra precautions during the COVID-19 pandemic, such as following social distancing guidelines, wearing masks, and washing hands regularly. Patients should also stay in close communication with their healthcare providers to manage their medications and monitor any changes in their heart rhythm.

The COVID-19 pandemic has shed light on the potential impact of the virus on the cardiovascular system, including the development or exacerbation of cardiac arrhythmias. Research suggests that COVID-19 can directly affect the heart, leading to inflammation, myocardial injury, and disturbances in the heart's electrical conduction system. Additionally, the systemic effects of the infection, such as inflammation, hypoxia, and electrolyte imbalances, can contribute to the occurrence of arrhythmias in COVID-19 patients. Cardiac arrhythmias have been observed in both mild and severe cases of COVID-19, and they can pose additional challenges in the management and treatment of affected individuals. Close monitoring of cardiac function, including continuous ECG monitoring in critical cases, is crucial to identify and manage arrhythmias promptly. Collaborative efforts between cardiologists and infectious disease specialists are essential to optimize the care of COVID-19 patients with cardiac arrhythmias and minimize the associated risks.

Chapter 13: Cardiac Arrhythmias and Sports

Participating in sports and physical activity is generally beneficial for heart health, but it can also increase the risk of cardiac arrhythmias in some individuals. Athletes and sports enthusiasts in West Bengal should be aware of the potential risks of cardiac arrhythmias and take steps to prevent them.

Athletes with a history of cardiac arrhythmias should undergo regular medical evaluations and may need to limit their physical activity or avoid certain types of sports. In addition, coaches and trainers should be trained to recognize the signs and symptoms of cardiac arrhythmias and know how to respond in case of an emergency.

Cardiac arrhythmias in sports present a unique challenge, as athletes strive for peak performance while managing their heart health. The intense physical demands of sports can trigger or exacerbate underlying arrhythmias, and certain arrhythmias can pose a risk of sudden cardiac events during athletic activities. It is crucial for athletes, coaches, and medical professionals to be aware of the potential risks, implement proper screening measures, and develop individualized management plans to ensure the safety and well-being of athletes with cardiac arrhythmias. Through a combination of medical supervision, appropriate training modifications, and timely interventions, athletes with cardiac arrhythmias can continue to pursue their passion for sports while prioritizing their cardiovascular health.

Chapter 14: Cardiac Arrhythmias in Children

Cardiac arrhythmias can occur in children of all ages, from infants to teenagers. In West Bengal, the most common types of cardiac arrhythmias in children include supraventricular tachycardia (SVT), Wolff-Parkinson-White syndrome (WPW), and long QT syndrome.

Diagnosing and treating cardiac arrhythmias in children requires specialized care from pediatric cardiologists and electrophysiologists. Treatment options may include medications, ablation, or implantable devices such as pacemakers or ICDs. Children with congenital heart defects may require surgery or other procedures to correct the underlying structural abnormalities.

Cardiac arrhythmias in children pose unique challenges due to their developing hearts and specific physiological considerations. While some arrhythmias in children may be benign and self-resolving, others can be more serious and require medical intervention. It is crucial for pediatricians and pediatric cardiologists to be vigilant in detecting and diagnosing cardiac arrhythmias in children, as early intervention can prevent potential complications. Treatment approaches may vary depending on the type and severity of the arrhythmia, ranging from medication to minimally invasive procedures or even implantation of devices like pacemakers or implantable cardioverter-defibrillators (ICDs). Close monitoring and follow-up care are essential to ensure optimal heart function and overall well-being for children affected by cardiac arrhythmias. Additionally, providing support and education to families is essential to empower them to manage their child's condition and navigate any lifestyle adjustments that may be necessary.

Chapter 15: Living with Cardiac Arrhythmias

Living with cardiac arrhythmias in West Bengal can be challenging, but there are many resources available to help patients and their families. Some of the ways to cope with cardiac arrhythmias include:

- Educating oneself about the condition and treatment options.

- Making lifestyle changes such as quitting smoking, eating a healthy diet, and staying physically active.

- Joining support groups or connecting with others who have similar experiences.

- Managing stress through relaxation techniques or counseling.

It is also important for patients with cardiac arrhythmias to stay in close communication with their healthcare providers and to follow their treatment plan to manage their symptoms and prevent complications.

Chapter 16: Advances in Cardiac Arrhythmia Research

Research into the causes and treatments of cardiac arrhythmias is ongoing in West Bengal and around the world. Some of the current areas of research include:

- Genetics: Studying the genetic factors that contribute to the development of cardiac arrhythmias.

- Stem cell therapy: Using stem cells to repair damaged heart tissue and restore normal heart function.

- Wearable technology: Developing wearable devices that can monitor heart rhythms and detect arrhythmias.

- Artificial intelligence: Using machine learning algorithms to analyze large datasets of heart rhythms and improve diagnosis and treatment.

These advances in research may lead to new and more effective treatments for cardiac arrhythmias in the future.

Chapter 17: Cardiac Arrhythmia Care in West Bengal

In West Bengal, there are many hospitals and healthcare providers that offer specialized care for cardiac arrhythmias. These include:

- Apollo Gleneagles Hospital in Kolkata, which has a dedicated department of cardiac electrophysiology and arrhythmia management.

- Fortis Hospital in Kolkata, which offers comprehensive care for all types of heart conditions, including cardiac arrhythmias.

- Medica Superspecialty Hospital in Kolkata, which has a team of expert cardiologists and electrophysiologists who provide advanced care for cardiac arrhythmias.

- Narayana Superspeciality Hospital in Howrah, which offers a range of diagnostic and treatment options for cardiac arrhythmias, including ablation and device implantation.

In addition to these hospitals, there are many clinics and healthcare providers throughout West Bengal that specialize in cardiac arrhythmia care. Patients should speak with their healthcare provider to determine the best option for their individual needs.

Chapter 18: Future Directions in Cardiac Arrhythmia Care

As technology and research continue to advance, the future of cardiac arrhythmia care in West Bengal looks promising. Some of the potential future directions include:

- Telemedicine: Using remote monitoring and telemedicine to improve access to care for patients in remote or underserved areas.

- Personalized medicine: Using genetic testing and individualized treatment plans to provide more targeted and effective care.

- Non-invasive treatments: Developing new non-invasive treatments for cardiac arrhythmias, such as focused ultrasound or magnetic fields.

- Integrated care: Integrating cardiac arrhythmia care with other aspects of heart health, such as hypertension management and lifestyle modifications.

These future directions hold great potential for improving the quality of care and outcomes for patients with cardiac arrhythmias in West Bengal and beyond.